MEDICAL AND HEALTH SCIENCE STATISTICS MADE EASY

2nd Edition

MEDICAL AND HEALTH SCIENCE STATISTICS MADE EASY

2nd Edition

Michael Harris
General Practitioner and Senior Lecturer in Medical Education, Bristol, UK

and

Gordon Taylor
Senior Lecturer in Medical Statistics, University of Bath, UK

JONES AND BARTLETT PUBLISHERS
Sudbury, Massachusetts
BOSTON   TORONTO   LONDON   SINGAPORE

World Headquarters
Jones and Bartlett
  Publishers
40 Tall Pine Drive
Sudbury, MA 01776
978-443-5000
info@jbpub.com
www.jbpub.com

Jones and Bartlett
  Publishers Canada
6339 Ormindale Way
Mississauga, Ontario
L5V 1J2
Canada

Jones and Bartlett
  Publishers International
Barb House, Barb Mews
London W6 7PA
United Kingdom

Jones and Bartlett's books and products are available through most bookstores and online booksellers. To contact Jones and Bartlett Publishers directly, call 800-832-0034, fax 978-443-8000, or visit our website www.jbpub.com.

Substantial discounts on bulk quantities of Jones and Bartlett's publications are available to corporations, professional associations, and other qualified organizations. For details and specific discount information, contact the special sales department at Jones and Bartlett via the above contact information or send an email to specialsales@jbpub.com.

Production Credits
Publisher: David Cella
Associate Editor: Maro Asadoorian
Senior Production Editor: Renée Sekerak
Production Editor: Tracey Chapman
Associate Marketing Manager: Lisa Gordon
Manufacturing and Inventory Control Supervisor: Amy Bacus
Composition: Publishers' Design & Production Services, Inc.
Cover Design: Kate Ternullo
Cover Image: © ihor_seamless/ShutterStock, Inc.
Printing and Binding: Malloy, Inc.
Cover Printing: Malloy, Inc.

Library of Congress Cataloging-in-Publication Data
Harris, Michael, 1956 Dec. 16–
  Medical and health science statistics made easy / Michael Harris and Gordon Taylor.
    p. cm.
  Includes bibliographical references and index.
  ISBN 978-0-7637-7265-9 (pbk.)
  1. Medical statistics.   I. Taylor, Gordon, 1970–   II. Title.
  RA409.H3728 2008
  610.72—dc22

                                                              2008049220

6048

Printed in the United States of America
12 11 10 09 08   10 9 8 7 6 5 4 3 2 1

CONTENTS

ABBREVIATIONS

ARR	absolute risk reduction
BMI	body mass index
BP	blood pressure
CI	confidence interval
df	degrees of freedom
HR	hazard ratio
IQR	inter-quartile range
LR	likelihood ratio
NNH	number needed to harm
NNT	number needed to treat
NPV	negative predictive value
P	probability
PPV	positive predictive value
RRR	relative risk reduction
SD	standard deviation
SE	side effect

PREFACE

This book is designed for healthcare students and professionals who need a basic knowledge of when common statistical terms are used and what they mean.

Whether you love or hate statistics, you need to have some understanding of the subject if you want to critically appraise a paper. To do this, you *do not* need to know how to do a statistical analysis. What you *do* need is to know why the test has been used and how to interpret the resulting figures.

This book does not assume that you have any prior statistical knowledge. However basic your mathematical or statistical knowledge, you will find that everything is clearly explained.

A few readers will find some of the sections ridiculously simplistic, others will find some bafflingly difficult. The "thumbs up" grading will help you pick out concepts that suit your level of understanding.

The "star" system is designed to help you pick out the most important concepts if you are short of time.

This book is also produced for those who may be asked about statistics in an exam. Pick out the "exam tips" sections if you are in a hurry.

You can test your understanding of what you have learned by working through extracts from original papers in the "Statistics at work" section.

ABOUT THE AUTHORS

Dr. Michael Harris, MB, BS, FRCGP, MMEd, is a General Practitioner and Senior Lecturer in Medical Education in Bristol, UK. He teaches nurses, medical students, and GP Registrars. Until recently he was an examiner for the MRCGP.

Dr. Gordon Taylor, PhD, MSc, BSc (Hons), is a Senior Lecturer in Medical Statistics at the University of Bath, UK. His main role is in the teaching, support, and supervision of healthcare professionals involved in noncommercial research.

FOREWORD

A love of statistics is, oddly, not what attracts most young people to a career in medicine and I suspect that many clinicians, like me, have at best a sketchy and incomplete understanding of this difficult subject.

Delivering modern, high-quality care to patients now relies increasingly on routine reference to scientific papers and journals, rather than traditional textbook learning. Acquiring the skills to appraise medical research papers is a daunting task. Realizing this, Michael Harris and Gordon Taylor have expertly constructed a practical guide for the busy clinician. One a practicing NHS doctor, the other a medical statistician with tremendous experience in clinical research, they have produced a unique handbook. It is short, readable, and useful, without becoming overly bogged down in the mathematical detail that frankly puts so many of us off the subject.

I commend this book to all healthcare professionals, general practitioners, and hospital specialists. It covers all the ground necessary to critically evaluate the statistical elements of medical research papers, in a friendly and approachable way. The scoring of each brief chapter in terms of usefulness and ease of comprehension will efficiently guide the busy practitioner through his or her reading.

Bill Irish
BSc, MB, BChir, DCH, DRCOG, MMEd, FRCGP
(Head of GP School, Severn Deanery, UK, and
Senior Examiner for the MRCGP(UK)).

HOW TO USE THIS BOOK

You can use this book in a number of ways.

If you want a statistics course

- Work through from start to finish for a complete course in commonly used medical statistics.

If you are in a hurry

- Choose the sections with the most stars to learn about the commonest statistical methods and terms.

- You may wish to start with these 5-star sections: percentages (page 7), mean (page 9), standard deviation (page 16), confidence intervals (page 20), and P values (page 24).

If you are daunted by statistics

- If you are bewildered every time someone tries to explain a statistical method, then pick out the sections with the most thumbs-up symbols to find the easiest and most basic concepts.

- You may want to start with percentages (page 7), mean (page 9), median (page 12), and mode (page 14), then move on to risk ratio (page 37), incidence, and prevalence (page 70).

If you are taking an exam

- The "Exam Tips" give you pointers to the topics which examiners like to ask about.

- You will find these in the following sections: mean (page 9), standard deviation (page 16), confidence intervals (page 20), *P* values (page 24), risk reduction and NNT (page 43), sensitivity, specificity, and predictive value (page 62), incidence and prevalence (page 70).

Test your understanding

- See how statistical methods are used in five extracts from real-life papers in the "Statistics at work" section (page 73).

- Work out which statistical methods have been used, why, and what the results mean. Then check your understanding in our commentary.

Glossary

- Use the glossary (page 93) as a quick reference for statistical words or phrases that you do not know.

Study advice

- Go through difficult sections when you are fresh and try not to cover too much at once.

- You may need to read some sections a couple of times before the meaning sinks in. You will find that the examples help you to understand the principles.

- We have tried to cut down the jargon as much as possible. If there is a word that you do not understand, check it out in the glossary.

HOW THIS BOOK IS DESIGNED

Every section uses the same series of headings to help you understand the concepts.

"How important is it?"

We noted how often statistical terms were used in 200 quantitative papers in mainstream medical journals. All the papers selected were published during the last year in the *British Medical Journal*, *The Lancet*, the *New England Journal of Medicine*, and the *Journal of the American Medical Association*.

We grouped the terms into concepts and graded them by how often they were used. This helped us to develop a star system for importance. We also took into account usefulness to readers. For example, "numbers needed to treat" are not often quoted but are fairly easy to calculate and useful in making treatment decisions.

✪✪✪✪✪   Concepts that are used in the majority of medical papers.

✪✪✪✪   Important concepts that are used in at least a third of papers.

✪✪✪   Less frequently used, but still of value in decision-making.

✪✪   Found in at least one in ten papers.

✪   Rarely used in medical journals.

How easy is it to understand?

We have found that the ability of healthcare professionals to understand statistical concepts varies more widely than their ability to understand anything else related to medicine. This ranges from those that have no difficulty learning how to understand regression to those that struggle with percentages.

One of the authors (not the statistician!) fell into the latter category. He graded each section by how easy it is to understand the concept.

👍👍👍👍👍   Even the most statistic-phobic will have little difficulty in understanding these sections.

👍👍👍👍   With a little concentration, most readers should be able to follow these concepts.

👍👍👍   Some readers will have difficulty following these. You may need to go over these sections a few times to be able to take them in.

👍👍   Quite difficult to understand. Only tackle these sections when you are fresh.

👍   Statistical concepts that are very difficult to grasp.

When is it used?

One thing you need to do if you're critically appraising a paper is check that the right statistical technique has been used. This part explains which statistical method should be used for what scenario.

What does it mean?

This explains the bottom line—what the results mean and what to look out for to help you interpret them.

Examples

Sometimes the best way to understand a statistical technique is to work through an example. Simple, fictitious examples are given to illustrate the principles and how to interpret them.

Watch out for ...

This includes more detailed explanation, tips, and common pitfalls.

Exam tips

Some topics are particularly popular with examiners because they test understanding and involve simple calculations. We have given tips on how to approach these concepts.

PERCENTAGES

How important are they?

✪✪✪✪✪   An understanding of percentages is probably the first and most important concept to understand in statistics!

How easy are they to understand?

👍👍👍👍👍   Percentages are easy to understand.

When are they used?

Percentages are mainly used in the tabulation of data in order to give the reader a scale on which to assess or compare the data.

What do they mean?

"Per cent" means per hundred, so a percentage describes a proportion of 100. For example 50% is 50 out of 100, or as a fraction ½. Other common percentages are 25% (25 out of 100 or ¼), 75% (75 out of 100 or ¾).

To calculate a percentage, divide the number of items or patients in the category by the total number in the group and multiply by 100.

EXAMPLE

Data were collected on 80 patients referred for heart transplantation. The researcher wanted to compare their ages. The data for age were put in "decade bands" and are shown in *Table 1*.

Table 1. Ages of 80 patients referred for heart transplantation

Years[a]	Frequency[b]	Percentage[c]
0–9	2	2.5
10–19	5	6.25
20–29	6	7.5
30–39	14	17.5
40–49	21	26.25
50–59	20	25
≥ 60	12	15
Total	80	100

[a] Years = decade bands;

[b] Frequency = number of patients referred;

[c] Percentage = percentage of patients in each decade band. For example, in the 30–39 age band there were 14 patients and we know the ages of 80 patients, so $\frac{14}{80} \times 100 = 17.5\%$.

Watch out for . . .

Authors can use percentages to hide the true size of the data. To say that 50% of a sample has a certain condition when there are only four people in the sample is clearly not providing the same level of information as 50% of a sample based on 400 people. So, percentages should be used as an additional help for the reader rather than replacing the actual data.

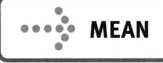 **MEAN**

Otherwise known as an arithmetic mean, or average.

How important is it?

✪✪✪✪✪ A mean appeared in 90% papers surveyed, so it is important to have an understanding of how it is calculated.

How easy is it to understand?

👍👍👍👍👍 One of the simplest statistical concepts to grasp. However, in most groups that we have taught there has been at least one person who admits not knowing how to calculate the mean, so we do not apologize for including it here.

When is it used?

It is used when the spread of the data is fairly similar on each side of the midpoint, for example, when the data are "normally distributed."

The "normal distribution" is referred to a lot in statistics. It's the symmetrical, bell-shaped distribution of data shown in *Fig. 1*.

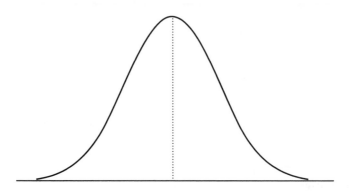

Fig. 1. The normal distribution. The dotted line shows the mean of the data.

What does it mean?

The mean is the sum of all the values, divided by the number of values.

EXAMPLE

Five women in a study on lipid-lowering agents are aged 52, 55, 56, 58, and 59 years.

Add these ages together:

$52 + 55 + 56 + 58 + 59 = 280$

Now divide by the number of women:

$\dfrac{280}{5} = 56$

So the mean age is 56 years.

Watch out for...

If a value (or a number of values) is a lot smaller or larger than the others, "skewing" the data, the mean will then not give a good picture of the typical value.

For example, if there is a sixth patient aged 92 in the study, then the mean age would be 62, even though only one woman is over 60 years old. In this case, the "median" may be a more suitable midpoint to use (see page 12).

A common multiple choice question is to ask the difference between mean, median (see page 12), and mode (see page 14)—make sure that you do not get confused between them.

●●●◦● MEDIAN

Sometimes known as the midpoint.

How important is it?

✪✪✪✪   It is given in over a half of mainstream papers.

How easy is it to understand?

👍👍👍👍   Even easier than the mean!

When is it used?

It is used to represent the average when the data are not symmetrical, for instance the "skewed" distribution in *Fig. 2*. Compare the shape of the graph with the normal distribution shown in *Fig. 1*.

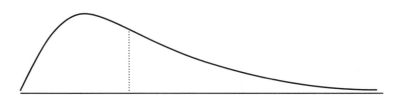

Fig. 2. A skewed distribution. The dotted line shows the median.

What does it mean?

It is the point that has half the values above, and half below.

EXAMPLE

Using the first example from page 10 of five patients aged 52, 55, 56, 58, and 59, the median age is 56, the same as the mean—half the women are older; half are younger.

However, in the second example with six patients aged 52, 55, 56, 58, 59, and 92 years, there are two "middle" ages, 56 and 58. The median is half-way between these, i.e., 57 years. This gives a better idea of the midpoint of this skewed data than the mean of 62.

Watch out for...

The median may be given with its interquartile range (IQR). The 1st quartile point has the ¼ of the data below it, the 3rd quartile point has the ¾ of the sample below it, so the IQR contains the middle ½ of the sample. This can be shown in a "box and whisker" plot.

EXAMPLE

A dietician measured the energy intake over 24 hours of 50 patients on a variety of wards. One ward had two patients that were "nil by mouth." The median was 12.2 megajoules, IQR 9.9 to 13.6. The lowest intake was 0; the highest was 16.7. This distribution is represented by the box and whisker plot in *Fig. 3*.

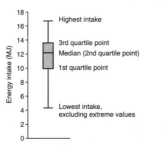

Fig. 3. Box and whisker plot of energy intake of 50 patients over 24 hours. The ends of the whiskers represent the maximum and minimum values, excluding extreme results like those of the two "nil by mouth" patients.

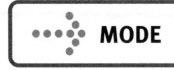 **MODE**

How important is it?

✖　　　　　　　Rarely quoted in papers and of limited value.

How easy is it to understand?

👍👍👍👍　An easy concept.

When is it used?

It is used when we need a label for the most frequently occurring event.

What does it mean?

The mode is the most common of a set of events.

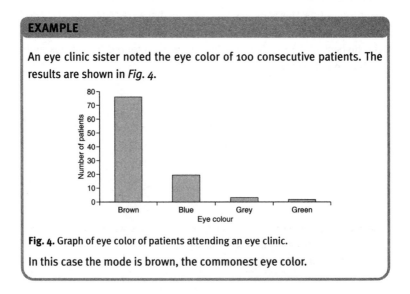

EXAMPLE

An eye clinic sister noted the eye color of 100 consecutive patients. The results are shown in *Fig. 4*.

Fig. 4. Graph of eye color of patients attending an eye clinic.

In this case the mode is brown, the commonest eye color.

You may see reference to a "bimodal distribution." Generally when this is mentioned in papers it is as a concept rather than from calculating the actual values, e.g., "The data appear to follow a bimodal distribution." See *Fig. 5* for an example of where there are two "peaks" to the data, i.e., a bimodal distribution.

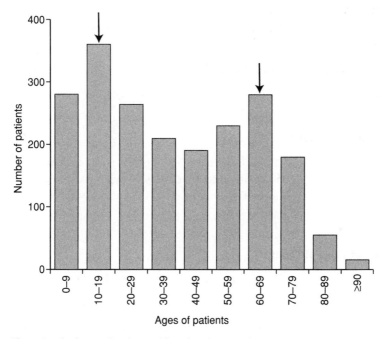

Fig. 5. Graph of ages of patients with asthma in a practice.

The arrows point to the modes at ages 10–19 and 60–69.

Bimodal data may suggest that two populations are present that are mixed together, so an average is not a suitable measure for the distribution.

STANDARD DEVIATION

How important is it?

✪✪✪✪✪ Quoted in two-thirds of papers, it is used as the basis of a number of statistical calculations.

How easy is it to understand?

👍👍👍 It is not an intuitive concept.

When is it used?

Standard deviation (SD) is used for data that are "normally distributed" (see page 9), to provide information on how much the data vary around their mean.

What does it mean?

SD indicates how much a set of values is spread around the average.

A range of one SD above and below the mean (abbreviated to ± 1 SD) includes 68.2% of the values.

± 2 SD includes 95.4% of the data.

± 3 SD includes 99.7%.

EXAMPLE

Let us say that a group of patients enrolling for a trial had a normal distribution for weight. The mean weight of the patients was 80 kg. For this group, the SD was calculated to be 5 kg.

1 SD below the average is 80 − 5 = 75 kg.

1 SD above the average is 80 + 5 = 85 kg.

± 1 SD will include 68.2% of the subjects, so 68.2% of patients will weigh between 75 and 85 kg.

95.4% will weigh between 70 and 90 kg (± 2 SD).

99.7% of patients will weigh between 65 and 95 kg (± 3 SD).

See how this relates to the graph of the data in *Fig. 6*.

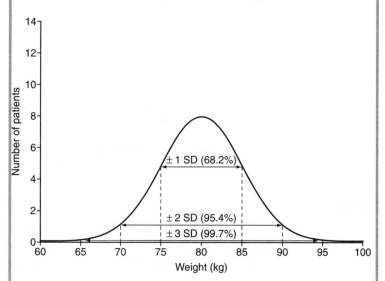

Fig. 6. Graph showing normal distribution of weights of patients enrolling in a trial with mean 80 kg, SD 5 kg.

If we have two sets of data with the same mean but different SDs, then the data set with the larger SD has a wider spread than the data set with the smaller SD.

For example, if another group of patients enrolling for the trial has the same mean weight of 80 kg but an SD of only 3, ± 1 SD will include 68.2% of the subjects, so 68.2% of patients will weigh between 77 and 83 kg (*Fig. 7*). Compare this with the example above.

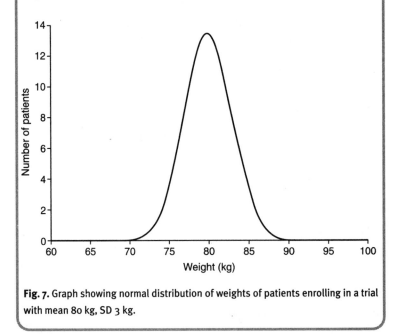

Fig. 7. Graph showing normal distribution of weights of patients enrolling in a trial with mean 80 kg, SD 3 kg.

Watch out for...

SD should only be used when the data have a normal distribution. However, means and SDs are often wrongly used for data that are not normally distributed.

A simple check for a normal distribution is to see if 2 SDs away from the mean are still within the possible range for the variable. For example, if we have some length of hospital stay data with a mean stay of 10 days and a SD of 8 days then:

mean − 2 × SD = 10 − 2 × 8 = 10 − 16 = −6 days.

This is clearly an impossible value for length of stay, so the data cannot be normally distributed. The mean and SDs are therefore not appropriate measures to use.

Good news—it is not necessary to know how to calculate the SD.

It *is* worth learning the figures above off by heart, so a reminder—

± 1 SD includes 68.2% of the data,

± 2 SD includes 95.4%,

± 3 SD includes 99.7%.

Keeping the "normal distribution" curve in *Fig. 6* in mind may help.

Examiners may ask what percentages of subjects are included in 1, 2, or 3 SDs from the mean. Again, try to memorize those percentages.

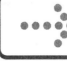 **CONFIDENCE INTERVALS**

How important are they?

✪✪✪✪✪   Important—given in three-quarters of papers.

How easy are they to understand?

👍👍   A difficult concept, but one in which a small amount of understanding will get you by without having to worry about the details.

When is it used?

Confidence intervals (CI) are typically used when, instead of simply wanting the mean value of a sample, we want a range that is likely to contain the true population value.

This "true value" is another tough concept—it is the mean value that we would get if we had data for the whole population.

What does it mean?

Statisticians can calculate a range (interval) in which we can be fairly sure (confident) that the "true value" lies.

For example, we may be interested in blood pressure (BP) reduction with antihypertensive treatment. From a sample of treated patients we can work out the mean change in BP.

However, this will only be the mean for our particular sample. If we took another group of patients, we would not expect to get exactly the same value because chance can also affect the change in BP.

The CI gives the range in which the true value (i.e. the mean change in BP if we treated an infinite number of patients) is likely to be.

EXAMPLES

The average systolic BP before treatment in study A, of a group of 100 hypertensive patients, was 170 mmHg. After treatment with the new drug the mean BP dropped by 20 mmHg.

If the 95% CI is 15–25, this means we can be 95% confident that the true effect of treatment is to lower the BP by 15–25 mmHg.

In study B, 50 patients were treated with the same drug, also reducing their mean BP by 20 mmHg, but with a wider 95% CI of −5 to +45. This CI includes zero (no change). This means there is more than a 5% chance that there was no true change in BP and that the drug was actually ineffective.

Watch out for...

The size of a CI is related to the sample size of the study. Larger studies usually have a narrower CI.

Where a few interventions, outcomes or studies are given it is difficult to visualize a long list of means and CIs. Some papers will show a chart to make it easier.

For example, "meta-analysis" is a technique for bringing together results from a number of similar studies to give one overall estimate of effect. Many meta-analyses compare the treatment effects from those studies by showing the mean changes and 95% CIs in a chart. An example is given in *Fig. 8*.

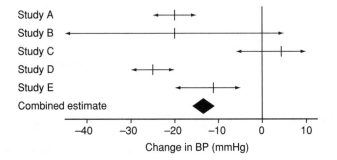

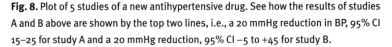

Fig. 8. Plot of 5 studies of a new antihypertensive drug. See how the results of studies A and B above are shown by the top two lines, i.e., a 20 mmHg reduction in BP, 95% CI 15–25 for study A and a 20 mmHg reduction, 95% CI −5 to +45 for study B.

The vertical axis does not have a scale. It is simply used to show the zero point on each CI line.

The statistician has combined the results of all five studies and calculated that the overall mean reduction in BP is 14 mmHg, CI 12–16. This is shown by the "combined estimate" diamond. See how combining a number of studies reduces the CI, giving a more accurate estimate of the true treatment effect.

The chart shown in *Fig. 8* is called a "Forest plot" or, more colloquially, a "blobbogram."

Standard deviation and confidence intervals—what is the difference? Standard deviation tells us about the variability (spread) in a sample.

The CI tells us the range in which the true value (the mean if the sample were infinitely large) is likely to be.

An exam question may give a chart similar to that in *Fig. 8* and ask you to summarize the findings. Consider:

- Which study showed the greatest change?

- Did all the studies show change in favor of the intervention?

- Were the changes statistically significant?

In the example above, study D showed the greatest change, with a mean BP drop of 25 mmHg.

Study C resulted in a mean increase in BP, though with a wide CI. The wide CI could be due to a low number of patients in the study.

The combined estimate of a mean BP reduction of 14 mmHg, 95% CI 12–16, is statistically significant.

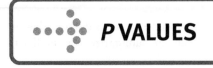

P VALUES

How important is it?

✪✪✪✪✪   A really important concept, P values are given in more than four out of five papers.

How easy is it to understand?

👍👍👍   Not easy, but worth persevering as it is used so frequently.

It is not important to know how the P value is derived—just to be able to interpret the result.

When is it used?

The P (probability) value is used when we wish to see how likely it is that a hypothesis is true. The hypothesis is usually that there is *no* difference between two treatments, known as the "null hypothesis."

What does it mean?

The P value gives the probability of any observed difference having happened by chance.

$P = 0.5$ means that the probability of the difference having happened by chance is 0.5 in 1, or 50:50.

$P = 0.05$ means that the probability of the difference having happened by chance is 0.05 in 1, i.e., 1 in 20.

It is the figure frequently quoted as being "statistically significant," i.e., unlikely to have happened by chance and therefore important. However, this is an arbitrary figure.

If we look at 20 studies, even if none of the treatments work, one of the studies is likely to have a *P* value of 0.05 and so appear significant!

The lower the *P* value, the less likely it is that the difference happened by chance and so the higher the significance of the finding.

$P = 0.01$ is often considered to be "highly significant." It means that the difference will only have happened by chance 1 in 100 times. This is unlikely, but still possible.

$P = 0.001$ means the difference will have happened by chance 1 in 1000 times, even less likely, but still just possible. It is usually considered to be "very highly significant."

EXAMPLES

Out of 50 new babies on average 25 will be girls, sometimes more, sometimes less.

Say there is a new fertility treatment and we want to know whether it affects the chance of having a boy or a girl. Therefore we set up a null hypothesis — that the treatment *does not* alter the chance of having a girl. Out of the first 50 babies resulting from the treatment, 15 are girls. We then need to know the probability that this just happened by chance, i.e., did this happen by chance or has the treatment had an effect on the sex of the babies?

The *P* value gives the probability that the null hypothesis is true.

The *P* value in this example is 0.007. Do not worry about how it was calculated; concentrate on what it means. It means the result would only have happened by chance in 0.007 in 1 (or 1 in 140) times if the treatment did not actually affect the sex of the baby. This is highly unlikely, so we can reject our hypothesis and conclude that the treatment probably *does* alter the chance of having a girl.

Try another example: Patients with minor illnesses were randomized to see either Dr. Smith or Dr. Jones. Dr. Smith ended up seeing 176 patients in the study, whereas Dr. Jones saw 200 patients (*Table 2*).

Table 2. Number of patients with minor illnesses seen by two GPs

	Dr. Jones ($n = 200$)[a]	Dr. Smith ($n = 176$)	P value	i.e., could have happened by chance
Patients satisfied with consultation (%)	186 (93)	168 (95)	0.4	Four times in 10 — possible
Mean (SD) consultation length (minutes)	16 (3.1)	6 (2.8)	<0.001	<One time in 1000 — very unlikely
Patients getting a prescription (%)	58 (29)	76 (43)	0.3	Three times in 10 — possible
Mean (SD) number of days off work	3.5 (1.3)	3.6 (1.3)	0.8	Eight times in 10 — probable
Patients needing a follow-up appointment (%)	46 (23)	72 (41)	0.05	Only one time in 20 — fairly unlikely

[a] $n = 200$ means that the total number of patients seen by Dr. Jones was 200.

Watch out for...

The "null hypothesis" is a concept that underlies this and other statistical tests.

The test method assumes (hypothesizes) that there is *no* (null) difference between the groups. The result of the test either supports or rejects that hypothesis.

The null hypothesis is generally the opposite of what we are actually interested in finding out. If we are interested in whether there is a difference between two treatments, then the null hypothesis would be that there is no difference and we would try to disprove this.

Try not to confuse statistical significance with clinical relevance. If a study is too small, the results are unlikely to be statistically significant even if the intervention actually works. Conversely, a large study may find a statistically significant difference that is too small to have any clinical relevance.

You may be given a set of *P* values and asked to interpret them. Remember that $P = 0.05$ is usually classed as "significant," $P = 0.01$ as "highly significant," and $P = 0.001$ as "very highly significant."

In the example above, only two of the sets of data showed a significant difference between the two GPs. Dr. Smith's consultations were very highly significantly shorter than those of Dr. Jones. Dr. Smith's follow-up rate was significantly higher than that of Dr. Jones.

_t_ TESTS AND OTHER PARAMETRIC TESTS

How important are they?

✪✪✪✪ Used in one in three papers, they are an important aspect of medical statistics.

How easy are they to understand?

👍 The details of the tests themselves are difficult to understand.

Thankfully, you do not need to know them. Just look for the _P_ value (see page 24) to see how significant the result is. Remember, the smaller the _P_ value, the smaller the chance that the "null hypothesis" is true.

When are they used?

Parametric statistics are used to compare samples of "normally distributed" data (see page 9). If the data do _not_ follow a normal distribution, these tests should not be used.

What do they mean?

A parametric test is any test that requires the data to follow a specific distribution, usually a normal distribution. Common parametric tests you will come across are the _t_ test and the χ^2 test.

Analysis of variance (ANOVA). This is a group of statistical techniques used to compare the means of two or more samples to see whether they come from the same population—the "null hypothesis." These techniques can also allow for independent variables, which may have an effect on the outcome.

Again, check out the *P* value.

t *test (also known as Student's* t). *t* tests are typically used to compare just two samples. They test the probability that the samples come from a population with the same mean value.

χ^2 *test.* A frequently used parametric test is the χ^2 test. It is covered separately (page 34).

EXAMPLE

Two hundred adults seeing an asthma nurse specialist were randomly assigned to either a new type of bronchodilator or placebo.

After 3 months, the peak flow rates in the treatment group had increased by a mean of 96 l/min (SD 58), and in the placebo group by 70 l/min (SD 52). The null hypothesis is that there is <u>no</u> difference between the bronchodilator and the placebo.

The *t* statistic is 11.14, resulting in a *P* value of 0.001. It is therefore very unlikely (1 in 1000 chance) that the null hypothesis is correct so we reject the hypothesis and conclude that the new bronchodilator is significantly better than the placebo.

Watch out for...

Parametric tests should only be used when the data follow a "normal" distribution. You may find reference to the "Kolmogorov Smirnov" test. This tests the hypothesis that the collected data are from a normal distribution and therefore assesses whether parametric statistics can be used.

Sometimes authors will say that they have "transformed" data and then analyzed them with a parametric test. This is quite legitimate—it is not cheating! For example, a skewed distribution might become normally distributed if the logarithm of the values is used.

MANN–WHITNEY AND OTHER NONPARAMETRIC TESTS

How important are they?

✪✪   Used in one in five papers.

How easy are they to understand?

👍   Nonparametric testing is difficult to understand.

However, you do not need to know the details of the tests. Look out for the *P* value (see page 24) to see how significant the results are. Remember, the smaller the *P* value, the smaller the chance that the "null hypothesis" is true.

When are they used?

Nonparametric statistics are used when the data are *not* normally distributed and so are not appropriate for "parametric" tests.

What do they mean?

Rather than comparing the values of the raw data, statisticians "rank" the data and compare the ranks.

EXAMPLE

Mann–Whitney U test. A GP introduced a nurse triage system into her practice. She was interested in finding out whether the age of the patients attending for triage appointments was different from that of patients who made emergency appointments with the GP.

Six hundred and forty-six patients saw the triage nurse and 532 patients saw the GP. The median age of the triaged patients was 50 years (1st quartile 40 years, 3rd quartile 54), for the GP it was 46 (22, 58). Note how the quartiles show an uneven distribution around the median, so the data cannot be normally distributed and a nonparametric test is appropriate. The graph in *Fig. 9* shows the ages of the patients seen by the nurse and confirms a skewed, rather than normal, distribution.

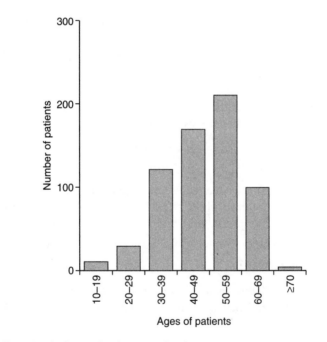

Fig. 9. Graph of ages of patients seen by triage nurse.

The statistician used a "Mann–Whitney U test" to test the hypothesis that there is no difference between the ages of the two groups. This gave a U value of 133 200 with a P value of <0.001. Ignore the actual U value but concentrate on the P value, which in this case suggests that the triage nurse's patients were very highly significantly older than those who saw the GP.

Watch out for...

The "Wilcoxon signed rank test" and "Kruskal Wallis" and "Friedman" tests are other nonparametric tests. Do not be put off by the names—go straight to the P value.

•••• ✚ CHI-SQUARED TEST

Usually written as χ^2 (for the test) or X^2 (for its value); Chi is pronounced as in sky without the s.

How important is it?

✪✪✪✪ A frequently used test of significance, given in a quarter of papers.

How easy is it to understand?

👍👍 Do not try to understand the X^2 value, just look at whether the result is significant.

When is it used?

It is a measure of the difference between actual and expected frequencies.

What does it mean?

The "expected frequency" is that there is no difference between the sets of results (the null hypothesis). In that case, the X^2 value would be zero.

The larger the actual difference between the sets of results, the greater the X^2 value. However, it is difficult to interpret the X^2 value by itself as it depends on the number of factors studied.

Statisticians make it easier for you by giving the P value (see page 24), giving you the likelihood there is no real difference between the groups.

So, do not worry about the actual value of X^2 but look at its P value.

EXAMPLES

A group of patients with bronchopneumonia were treated with either amoxicillin or erythromycin. The results are shown in *Table 3*.

Table 3. Comparison of effect of treatment of bronchopneumonia with amoxicillin or erythromycin

| | Type of antibiotic given | | |
	Amoxicillin	Erythromycin	Total
Improvement at 5 days	144 (60%)	160 (67%)	304 (63%)
No improvement at 5 days	96 (40%)	80 (33%)	176 (37%)
Total	240 (100%)	240 (100%)	480 (100%)
	$X^2 = 2.3$; $P = 0.13$		

A table like this is known as a "contingency table" or "two-way table."

First, look at the table to get an idea of the differences between the effects of the two treatments.

Remember, do not worry about the X^2 value itself but see whether it is significant. In this case P is 0.13, so the difference in treatments is not statistically significant.

Watch out for...

Some papers will also give the "degrees of freedom" (df), for example, $X^2 = 2.3$; df 1; $P = 0.13$. See page 98 for an explanation. This is used with the X^2 value to work out the P value.

Other tests you may find. Instead of the χ^2 test, "Fisher's exact test" is sometimes used to analyze contingency tables. Fisher's test is the best choice as it always gives the exact P value, particularly where the numbers are small.

The χ^2 test is simpler for statisticians to calculate but gives only an approximate P value and is inappropriate for small samples. Statisticians may apply "Yates' continuity correction" or other adjustments to the χ^2 test to improve the accuracy of the P value.

The "Mantel Haenszel test" is an extension of the χ^2 test that is used to compare several two-way tables.

RISK RATIO

Often referred to as relative risk.

How important is it?

✪✪✪   Used in one in six papers.

How easy is it to understand?

👍👍👍👍   Risk is a relatively intuitive concept that we encounter every day, but interpretation of risk (especially low risk) is often inconsistent. The risk of death while traveling to the shops to buy a lottery ticket can be higher than the risk of winning the jackpot!

When is it used?

Relative risk is used in "cohort studies," prospective studies that follow a group (cohort) over a period of time and that investigate the effect of a treatment or risk factor.

What does it mean?

First, risk itself. *Risk* is the probability that an event will happen. It is calculated by dividing the number of events by the number of people at risk.

One boy is born for every two births, so the probability (risk) of giving birth to a boy is

$$\frac{1}{2} = 0.5$$

If one in every 100 patients suffers a side-effect from a treatment, the risk is

$$\frac{1}{100} = 0.01$$

Compare this with odds (page 40).

Now, risk *ratios*. These are calculated by dividing the risk in the treated or exposed group by the risk in the control or unexposed group.

A risk ratio of one indicates no difference in risk between the groups.

If the risk ratio of an event is >1, the rate of that event is increased compared to controls.

If <1, the rate of that event is reduced.

Risk ratios are frequently given with their 95% CIs— if the CI for a risk ratio *does not* include one (no difference in risk), it is statistically significant.

EXAMPLES

A cohort of 1000 regular football players and 1000 nonfootball players were followed to see if playing football was significant in the injuries that they received.

After 1 year of follow-up, there had been 12 broken legs in the football players and only four in the nonfootball players.

The *risk* of a football player breaking a leg was therefore 12/1000 or 0.012. The risk of a nonfootball player breaking a leg was 4/1000 or 0.004.

The risk *ratio* of breaking a leg was therefore 0.012/0.004, which equals three. The 95% CI was calculated to be 0.97 to 9.41. As the CI includes the value 1, we cannot exclude the possibility that there was no difference in the risk of football players and nonfootball players breaking a leg. However, given these results, further investigation would clearly be warranted.

ODDS RATIO

How important is it?

✪✪✪✪   Used in a third of papers.

How easy is it to understand?

👍👍   Odds are difficult to understand. Just aim to understand what the ratio means.

When is it used?

Used by epidemiologists in studies looking for factors that do harm, it is a way of comparing patients who already have a certain condition (cases) with patients who do not (controls)—a "case–control study."

What does it mean?

First, *odds*. Odds are calculated by dividing the number of times an event happens by the number of times it does not happen.

One boy is born for every two births, so the odds of giving birth to a boy are 1:1 (or 50:50) = $\frac{1}{1}$ = 1

If one in every 100 patients suffers a side-effect from a treatment, the odds are

1:99 = $\frac{1}{99}$ = 0.0101

Compare this with risk (page 37).

Next, odds *ratios*. They are calculated by dividing the odds of having been exposed to a risk factor by the odds in the control group.

An odds ratio of 1 indicates no difference in risk between the groups, i.e., the odds in each group are the same.

If the odds ratio of an event is >1, the rate of that event is increased in patients who have been exposed to the risk factor.

If <1, the rate of that event is reduced.

Odds ratios are frequently given with their 95% CI— if the CI for an odds ratio *does not* include 1 (no difference in odds), it is statistically significant.

EXAMPLES

A group of 100 patients with knee injuries, "cases," was matched for age and sex to 100 patients who did not have injured knees, "controls."

In the cases, 40 skied and 60 did not, giving the *odds* of being a skier for this group of 40:60 or 0.66.

In the controls, 20 patients skied and 80 did not, giving the odds of being a skier for the control group of 20:80 or 0.25.

We can therefore calculate the odds *ratio* as 0.66/0.25 = 2.64. The 95% CI is 1.41 to 5.02.

If you cannot follow the maths, do not worry! The odds ratio of 2.64 means that the number of skiers in the cases is greater than the number of skiers in the controls, and as the CI does not include 1 (no difference in risk), this is statistically significant. Therefore, we can conclude that skiers are more likely to get a knee injury than nonskiers.

Watch out for...

Authors may give the percentage *change* in the odds ratio rather than the odds ratio itself. In the example above, the odds ratio of 2.64 means the same as a 164% increase in the odds of injured knees among skiers.

Odds ratios are often interpreted by the reader in the same way as risk ratios. This is reasonable when the odds are low, but for common events the odds and the risks (and therefore their ratios) will give very different values. For example, the odds of giving birth to a boy are 1, whereas the risk is 0.5. However, in the side-effect example given above the odds are 0.0101, a similar value to the risk of 0.01. For this reason, if you are looking at a case-control study, check that the authors have used odds ratios rather than risk ratios.

RISK REDUCTION AND NUMBERS NEEDED TO TREAT

How important are they?

Although only quoted in less than 5% of papers, they are helpful in trying to work out how worthwhile a treatment is in clinical practice.

How easy are they to understand?

"Relative risk reduction" (RRR) and "absolute risk reduction" (ARR) need some concentration. "Numbers needed to treat" (NNT) are pretty intuitive, useful, and not too difficult to work out for yourself.

When are they used?

They are used when an author wants to know how often a treatment works, rather than just whether it works.

What do they mean?

ARR is the difference between the event rate in the intervention group and that in the control group. It is also the reciprocal of the NNT and is usually given as a percentage, i.e., $ARR = \dfrac{100}{NNT}$.

NNT is the number of patients who need to be treated for one to get benefit.

RRR is the proportion by which the intervention reduces the event rate.

EXAMPLES

One hundred women with vaginal candida were given an oral antifungal; 100 were given placebo. They were reviewed 3 days later. The results are given in *Table 4*.

Table 4. Results of placebo-controlled trial of oral antifungal agent

Given antifungal		Given placebo	
Improved	No improvement	Improved	No improvement
80	20	60	40

ARR = improvement rate in the intervention group − improvement rate in the control group = 80% − 60% = 20%

$$NNT = \frac{100}{ARR} = \frac{100}{20} = 5$$

So five women have to be treated for one to get benefit.

The incidence of candidiasis was reduced from 40% with placebo to 20% with treatment, i.e., by half.

Thus, the RRR is 50%.

In another trial young men were treated with an expensive lipid-lowering agent. Five years later the death rate from ischaemic heart disease (IHD) is recorded. See *Table 5* for the results.

Table 5. Results of placebo-controlled trial of Cleverstatin

Given Cleverstatin		Given placebo	
Survived	Died	Survived	Died
998 (99.8%)	2 (0.2%)	996 (99.6%)	4 (0.4%)

ARR = improvement rate in the intervention group − improvement rate in the control group = 99.8% − 99.6% = 0.2%

$$NNT = \frac{100}{ARR} = \frac{100}{0.2} = 500$$

So 500 men have to be treated for 5 years for one to survive who would otherwise have died.

The incidence of death from IHD is reduced from 0.4% with placebo to 0.2% with treatment – i.e., by half.

Thus, the RRR is 50%.

The RRR and NNT from the same study can have opposing effects on prescribing habits. The RRR of 50% in this example sounds fantastic. However, thinking of it in terms of an NNT of 500 might sound less attractive: for every life saved, 499 patients had unnecessary treatment for 5 years.

Watch out for...

Usually the necessary percentages are given in the abstract of the paper. Calculating the ARR is easy: subtract the percentage that improved without treatment from the percentage that improved with treatment.

Again, dividing that figure into 100 gives the NNT.

With an NNT you need to know:

(a) What treatment?

- What are the side-effects?

- What is the cost?

(b) For how long?

(c) To achieve what?

- How serious is the event you are trying to avoid?

- How easy is it to treat if it happens?

For treatments, the lower the NNT the better—but look at the context.

(a) NNT of 10 for treating a sore throat with expensive blundamycin

- not attractive

(b) NNT of 10 for prevention of death from leukaemia with a nontoxic chemotherapy agent

- worthwhile

Expect NNTs for prophylaxis to be much larger. For example, an immunization may have an NNT in the thousands but still be well worthwhile.

Numbers needed to harm (NNH) may also be important.

$$NNH = \frac{100}{(\% \text{ on treatment that had SEs}) - (\% \text{ not on treatment that had SEs})}$$

In the example above, 6% of those on cleverstatin had peptic ulceration as opposed to 1% of those on placebo.

$$NNH = \frac{100}{6 - 1} = \frac{100}{5} = 20$$

i.e., for every 20 patients treated, one peptic ulcer was caused.

You may see ARR and RRR given as a proportion instead of a percentage. So, an ARR of 20% is the same as an ARR of 0.2.

Be prepared to calculate RRR, ARR, and NNT from a set of results. You may find that it helps to draw a simple table like *Table 5* and work from there.

CORRELATION

How important is it?

✪✪   Only used in 15% of medical papers.

How easy is it to understand?

👍👍👍

When is it used?

Where there is a linear relationship between two variables, there is said to be a correlation between them. Examples are height and weight in children, or socioeconomic class and mortality.

The *strength* of that relationship is given by the "correlation coefficient."

What does it mean?

The correlation coefficient is usually denoted by the letter "r" for example $r = 0.8$.

A *positive* correlation coefficient means that as one variable is increasing the value for the other variable is also increasing—the line on the graph slopes up from left to right. Height and weight have a positive correlation: children get heavier as they grow taller.

A *negative* correlation coefficient means that as the value of one variable goes up the value for the other variable goes down—the graph slopes down from left to right. Higher socioeconomic class is associated with a lower mortality, giving a negative correlation between the two variables.

If there is a perfect relationship between the two variables then $r = 1$ (if a positive correlation) or $r = -1$ (if a negative correlation).

If there is no correlation at all (the points on the graph are completely randomly scattered) then $r = 0$.

The following is a good rule of thumb when considering the size of a correlation:

$r = 0$–0.2 :   very low and probably meaningless.

$r = 0.2$–0.4 :   a low correlation that might warrant further investigation.

$r = 0.4$–0.6 :   a reasonable correlation.

$r = 0.6$–0.8 :   a high correlation.

$r = 0.8$–1.0 :   a very high correlation. Possibly too high! Check for errors or other reasons for such a high correlation.

This guide also applies to negative correlations.

Examples

A nurse wanted to be able to predict the laboratory HbA_{1c} result (a measure of blood glucose control) from the fasting blood glucoses that she measured in her clinic. On 12 consecutive diabetic patients, she noted the fasting glucose and simultaneously drew blood for HbA_{1c}. She compared the pairs of measurements and drew the graph in *Fig. 10*.

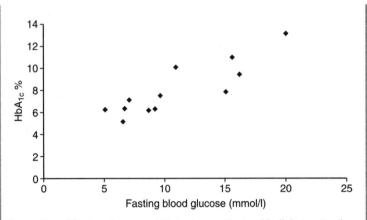

Fig. 10. Plot of fasting glucose and HbA$_{1c}$ in 12 patients with diabetes. For these results $r = 0.88$, showing a very high correlation.

A graph like this is known as a "scatter plot."

An occupational therapist developed a scale for measuring physical activity and wondered how much it correlated to Body Mass Index (BMI) in 12 of her adult patients. *Fig. 11* shows how they related.

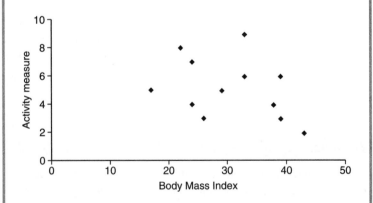

Fig. 11. BMI and activity measure in 12 adult patients.

In this example, $r = -0.34$, indicating a low correlation. The fact that the r value is negative shows that the correlation is negative, indicating that patients with a higher level of physical activity tended to have a lower BMI.

Watch out for...

Correlation tells us how strong the association between the variables is, but does not tell us about cause and effect in that relationship.

The "Pearson correlation coefficient," Pearson's r, is used if the values are sampled from "normal" populations (page 9). Otherwise the "Spearman rank correlation coefficient" is used. However, the interpretation of the two is the same.

Where the author shows the graph, you can get a good idea from the scatter as to how strong the relationship is without needing to know the r value.

Authors often give P values with correlations; however, take care when interpreting them. Although a correlation needs to be significant, we need also to consider the size of the correlation. If a study is sufficiently large, even a small clinically unimportant correlation will be highly significant.

R^2 is sometimes given. As it is the square of the r value, and squares are always positive, you cannot use it to tell whether the graph slopes up or down.

What it *does* tell you is how much of the variation in one value is caused by the other.

In *Fig. 10*, $r = 0.88$. $R^2 = 0.88 \times 0.88 = 0.77$. This means that 77% of the variation in HbA_{1c} is related to the variation in fasting glucose.

Again, the closer the R^2 value is to 1, the higher the correlation.

It is very easy for authors to compare a large number of variables using correlation and only present the ones that happen to be significant. So, check to make sure there is a plausible explanation for any significant correlations.

Also bear in mind that a correlation only tells us about linear (straight line) relationships between variables. Two variables may be strongly related but not in a straight line, giving a low correlation coefficient.

REGRESSION

How important is it?

✪✪✪   Regression analysis is used in a half of papers.

How easy is it to understand?

👍👍   The idea of trying to fit a line through a set of points to make the line as representative as possible is relatively straightforward. However, the mathematics involved in fitting regression models are more difficult to understand.

When is it used?

Regression analysis is used to find how one set of data relates to another.

This can be particularly helpful for instances in which we want to use one measure as a proxy for another—for example, a near-patient test as a proxy for a lab test.

What does it mean?

A regression line is the "best fit" line through the data points on a graph.

The regression coefficient gives the "slope" of the graph, in that it gives the change in value of one outcome, per unit change in the other.

EXAMPLE

Consider the graph shown in *Fig. 10* (page 50). A statistician calculated the line that gave the "best fit" through the scatter of points, shown in *Fig. 12*.

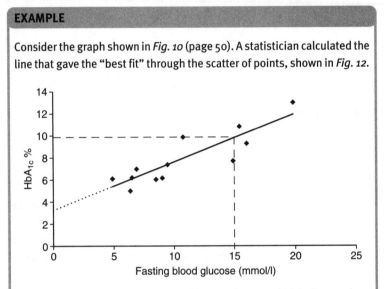

Fig. 12. Plot with linear regression line of fasting glucose and HbA_{1c} in 12 patients with diabetes.

The line is called a "regression line."

To predict the HbA_{1c} for a given blood glucose a nurse could simply plot it on the graph, as where a fasting glucose of 15 predicts an HbA_{1c} of 9.95%.

This can also be done mathematically. The slope and position of the regression line can be represented by the "regression equation":

$HbA_{1c} = 3.2 + (0.45 \times \text{blood glucose})$.

The 0.45 figure gives the *slope* of the graph and is called the "regression coefficient."

The "regression constant" that gives the *position* of the line on the graph is 3.2: it is the point where the line crosses the vertical axis.

Try this with a glucose of 15:

$HbA_{1c} = 3.2 + (0.45 \times 15) = 3.2 + 6.75 = 9.95\%$

This regression equation can be applied to any regression line. It is represented by:

$y = a + bx$

To predict the value y (value on the vertical axis of the graph) from the value x (on the horizontal axis), b is the regression coefficient and a is the constant.

Other values sometimes given with regression

You may see other values quoted. The regression coefficient and constant can be given with their "standard errors." These indicate the accuracy that can be given to the calculations. Do not worry about the actual value of these but look at their P values. The lower the P value, the greater the significance.

The R^2 value may also be given. This represents the amount of the variation in the data that is explained by the regression. In our example the R^2 value is 0.77. This is stating that 77% of the variation in the HbA_{1c} result is accounted for by variation in the blood glucose.

Other types of regression

The example above is a "linear regression," as the line that best fits the points is straight.

Other forms of regression include:

Logistic regression. This is used for instances in which each case in the sample can only belong to one of two groups (e.g., having disease or not) with the outcome as the probability that a case belongs to one group rather than the other.

Poisson regression. Poisson regression is mainly used to study waiting times or time between rare events.

Cox proportional hazards regression model. The Cox regression model (page 60) is used in survival analysis in which the outcome is time until a certain event.

Watch out for...

Regression should not be used to make predictions outside of the range of the original data. In the example above, we can only make predictions from blood glucoses that are between 5 and 20.

Regression or correlation?

Regression and correlation are easily confused.

Correlation measures the *strength* of the association between variables.

Regression *quantifies* the association. It should only be used if one of the variables is thought to precede or cause the other.

SURVIVAL ANALYSIS: LIFE TABLES AND KAPLAN–MEIER PLOTS

How important are they?

✪✪✪   Survival analysis techniques are used in 20% of papers.

How easy are they to understand?

👍👍👍   Life tables are difficult to interpret. Luckily, most papers make it easy for you by showing the resulting plots—these graphs give a good visual feel of what has happened to a population over time.

When are they used?

Survival analysis techniques are concerned with representing the time until a single event occurs. That event is often death, but it could be any other single event, for example, time until discharge from hospital.

Survival analysis techniques are able to deal with situations in which the end event has not happened in every patient or when information on a case is only known for a limited duration—known as "censored" observations.

What do they mean?

Life table. A life table is a table of the proportion of patients surviving over time.

Life table methods look at the data at a number of fixed time points and calculate the survival rate at those times. The most commonly used method is Kaplan–Meier.

Kaplan–Meier

The Kaplan–Meier approach recalculates the survival rate when an end event (e.g., death) occurs in the data set, i.e., when a change happens rather than at fixed intervals.

This is usually represented as a "survival plot." *Fig. 13* shows a fictitious example.

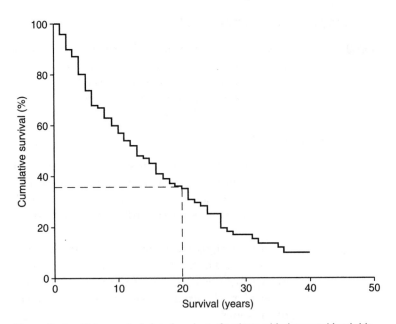

Fig. 13. Kaplan–Meier survival plot of a cohort of patients with rheumatoid arthritis.

The dashed line shows that at 20 years, 36% of this group of patients were still alive.

Watch out for...

Life tables and Kaplan–Meier survival estimates are also used to compare survival between groups. The plots make any difference between survival in two groups beautifully clear. *Fig. 14* shows the same group of patients as above but compares survival for men and women.

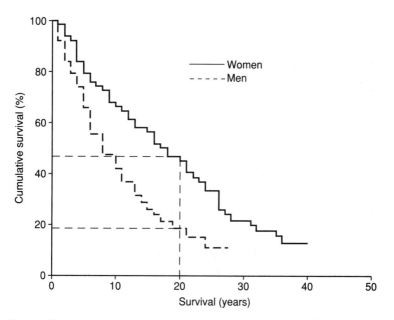

Fig. 14. Kaplan–Meier survival plot comparing men and women with rheumatoid arthritis.

In this example 46% of women were still alive at 20 years but only 18% of men.

The test to compare the survival between these two groups is called the "log rank test." Its *P* value will tell you how significant the result of the test is.

THE COX REGRESSION MODEL

Also known as the proportional hazards survival model.

How important is it?

✪✪   It appeared in a quarter of papers.

How easy is it to understand?

👍👍   Just aim to understand the end result—the "hazard ratio" (HR).

When is it used?

The Cox regression model is used to investigate the relationship between an event (usually death) and possible explanatory variables, for instance, smoking status or weight.

What does it mean?

The Cox regression model provides us with estimates of the effect that different factors have on the time until the end event.

As well as considering the significance of the effect of different factors (e.g., how much shorter male life expectancy is compared to that of women), the model can give us an estimate of life expectancy for an individual.

The "HR" is the ratio of the hazard (chance of something harmful happening) of an event in one group of observations divided by the hazard of an event in another group. An HR of 1 means the risk is 1 × that of the second group, i.e., the same. An HR of 2 implies twice the risk.

EXAMPLE

The Cox regression model shows us the effect of being in one group compared with another.

Using the rheumatoid arthritis cohort on page 58, we can calculate the effect that gender has on survival. *Table 6* gives the results of a Cox model estimate of the effect.

Table 6. Cox model estimate of the effect of sex on survival in a cohort of patients with rheumatoid arthritis

Parameter	HR[a] (95% CI)[b]	df [c]	P value[d]
Sex (Male)	1.91 (1.21 to 3.01)	1	<0.05

[a] The HR of 1.91 means that the risk of death in any particular time period for men was 1.91 times that for women.

[b] This CI means we can be 95% confident that the true HR is between 1.21 and 3.01.

[c] Degrees of freedom—see glossary, page 98.

[d] The P value of <0.05 suggests that the result is significant.

SENSITIVITY, SPECIFICITY, AND PREDICTIVE VALUE

How important are they?

✪✪✪   They are discussed in 40% of papers, so a working knowledge is important in interpreting papers that study screening.

How easy are they to understand?

👍👍👍   The tables themselves are fairly easy to understand. However, there is a bewildering array of information that can be derived from them.

To avoid making your head spin, do not read this section until you are feeling fresh. You may need to go over it a few days running until it is clear in your mind.

When are they used?

They are used to analyze the value of screening or tests.

What do they mean?

Think of any screening test for a disease. For each patient:

- the disease itself may be present or absent;

- the test result may be positive or negative.

We need to know how useful the test is.

The results can be put in the "two-way table" shown in *Table 7*. Try working through it.

Table 7. Two-way table

		Disease:	
		Present	Absent
Test result:	Positive	A	B (False positive)
	Negative	C (False negative)	D

Sensitivity. If a patient has the disease, we need to know how often the test will be positive, i.e., "positive in disease."

This is calculated from: $\dfrac{A}{A + C}$

This is the rate of pick-up of the disease in a test, and is called the *Sensitivity*.

Specificity. If the patient is in fact healthy, we want to know how often the test will be negative, i.e., "negative in health."

This is given by: $\dfrac{D}{D + B}$

This is the rate at which a test can exclude the possibility of the disease and is known as the *Specificity*.

Positive Predictive Value. If the test result is positive, what is the likelihood that the patient will have the condition?

Look at: $\dfrac{A}{A + B}$

This is known as the *Positive Predictive Value* (PPV).

Negative Predictive Value. If the test result is negative, what is the likelihood that the patient will be healthy?

Here we use: $\dfrac{D}{D+C}$

This is known as the *Negative Predictive Value* (NPV).

In a perfect test, the sensitivity, specificity, PPV, and NPV would each have a value of 1. The lower the value (the nearer to zero), the less useful the test is in that respect.

EXAMPLES

Confused? Try working through an example.

Imagine a blood test for gastric cancer, tried out on 100 patients admitted with haematemesis. The actual presence or absence of gastric cancers was diagnosed from endoscopic findings and biopsy. The results are shown in *Table 8.*

Table 8. Two-way table for blood test for gastric cancer

		Gastric cancer:	
		Present	Absent
Blood result:	Positive	20	30
	Negative	5	45

$\text{Sensitivity} = \dfrac{20}{20+5} = \dfrac{20}{25} = 0.8$

If the gastric cancer is present, there is an 80% (0.8) chance of the test picking it up.

$\text{Specificity} = \dfrac{45}{30+45} = \dfrac{45}{75} = 0.6$

If there is no gastric cancer, there is a 60% (0.6) chance of the test being negative—but 40% will have a false-positive result.

$$PPV = \frac{20}{20 + 30} = \frac{20}{50} = 0.4$$

There is a 40% (0.4) chance that, if the test is positive, the patient actually has gastric cancer.

$$NPV = \frac{45}{45 + 5} = \frac{45}{50} = 0.9$$

There is a 90% (0.9) chance that, if the test is negative, the patient does not have gastric cancer. However, there is still a 10% chance of a false negative, i.e., that the patient does have gastric cancer.

Watch out for...

One more test to know about.

The "Likelihood Ratio" (LR) is the likelihood that the test result would be expected in a patient with the condition compared to the likelihood that that same result would be expected in a patient without the condition.

To calculate the LR, divide the sensitivity by (1 – specificity).

Head spinning again? Try using the example above to calculate the LR for a positive result.

$$LR = \frac{\text{sensitivity}}{(1 - \text{specificity})} = \frac{0.8}{1 - 0.6} = \frac{0.8}{0.4} = 2$$

In this example, LR for a positive result = 2. This means that if the test is positive in a patient, that patient is twice as likely to have gastric cancer than not have it.

Tip: Invent an imaginary screening or diagnostic test of your own, fill the boxes in, and work out the various values. Then change the results to make the test a lot less or more effective and see how it affects the values.

One thing you may notice is that in a rare condition, even a diagnostic test with a very high sensitivity may result in a low PPV.

If you are still feeling confused, you are in good company. Many colleagues far brighter than us admit that they get confused over sensitivity, PPV, etc.

Try copying the following summary into your diary and refer to it when reading a paper:

- **Sensitivity:** How often the test is positive if the patient has the disease.

- **Specificity:** If the patient is healthy, how often the test will be negative.

- **PPV:** If the test is positive, the likelihood that the patient has the condition.

- **NPV:** If the test is negative, the likelihood that the patient will be healthy.

- **LR:** If the test is positive, how much more likely the patient is to have the disease than not have it.

Examiners love to give a set of figures that you can turn into a two-way table and ask you to calculate sensitivity, PPV, etc. from them. Keep practicing until you are comfortable at working with these values.

LEVEL OF AGREEMENT AND KAPPA

Kappa is often seen written as κ.

How important is it?

✪　　　Not often used.

How easy is it to understand?

👍👍👍

When is it used?

It is a comparison of how well people or tests agree and is used when data can be put into ordered categories.

Typically, it is used to look at how accurately a test can be repeated.

What does it mean?

The kappa value can vary from zero to 1.

A κ of zero means that there is no significant agreement—no more than would have been expected by chance.

A κ of 0.5 or more is considered a good agreement; a value of 0.7 shows very good agreement.

A κ of 1 means that there is perfect agreement.

EXAMPLE

If the same cervical smear slides are examined by the cytology departments of two hospitals and $\kappa = 0.3$, it suggests that there is little agreement between the two laboratories.

Watch out for...

Kappa can be used to analyze cervical smear results because they can be ordered into separate categories, e.g., CIN 1, CIN 2, CIN 3—so-called "ordinal data." When the variable that is being considered is continuous, for example blood glucose readings, the "intraclass correlation coefficient" should be used (see glossary).

OTHER CONCEPTS

Multiple testing adjustment

Importance: ✪
Ease of understanding: 👍👍

One fundamental principle of statistics is that we accept there is a chance we will come to the wrong conclusion. If we reject a null hypothesis with a P value of 0.05, then there is still the 5% possibility that we should not have rejected the hypothesis and therefore a 5% chance that we have come to the wrong conclusion.

If we do lots of testing then this chance of making a mistake will be present each time we do a test, and therefore the more tests we do, the greater the chances of drawing the wrong conclusion.

Multiple testing adjustment techniques therefore adjust the P value to keep the overall chance of coming to the wrong conclusion at a certain level (usually 5%).

The most commonly used method is the "Bonferroni" adjustment.

1- and 2-tailed tests

Importance: ✪
Ease of understanding: 👍

When trying to reject a "null hypothesis" (page 27), we are generally interested in two possibilities: either we can reject it because the new treatment is better than the current one or because it is worse. By allowing the null hypothesis to be rejected from either direction we are performing a "two-tailed test"—we are rejecting it when the result is in either "tail" of the test distribution.

Occasionally, there are situations in which we are only interested in rejecting a hypothesis if the new treatment is worse that the current one but not if it is better. This would be better analyzed with a one-tailed test. However, be very sceptical of one-tailed tests. A *P* value that is not quite significant on a two-tailed test may become significant if a one-tailed test is used. Authors have been known to use this to their advantage!

Incidence

Importance: ✪✪✪✪
Ease of understanding: 👍👍👍👍

The number of **new** cases of a condition **over a given time** as a percentage of the population.

Example: Each year 15 people in a practice of 1000 patients develop Brett's palsy.

$$\frac{15}{1000} \times 100 = \text{yearly incidence of } 1.5\%$$

Prevalence (= Point Prevalence Rate)

Importance ✪✪✪✪
Ease of understanding: 👍👍👍👍

The **existing** number of cases of a condition at **a single point in time** as a percentage of the population.

Example: At the time of a study, 90 people in a practice of 1000 patients were suffering from Brett's palsy (15 diagnosed in the last year plus 75 diagnosed in previous years).

$$\frac{90}{1000} \times 100 = \text{a prevalence of 9\%}$$

With chronic diseases like the fictitious Brett's palsy, the incidence will be lower than the prevalence—each year's new diagnoses swell the number of existing cases.

With short-term illnesses the opposite may be true. 75% of a population may have a cold each year (incidence), but at any moment only 2% are actually suffering (prevalence).

 Check that you can explain the difference between incidence and prevalence.

Power

Importance: ✪✪
Ease of understanding: 👍👍👍

The power of a study is the probability that it would detect a statistically significant difference.

If the difference expected is 100% cure compared with 0% cure with previous treatments, a very small study would have sufficient power to detect that.

However if the expected difference is much smaller, e.g., 1%, then a small study would be unlikely to have enough power to produce a result with statistical significance.

Bayesian statistics

Importance: ✪
Ease of understanding: 👍

Bayesian analysis is not often used. It is a totally different statistical approach to the classical, "frequentist" statistics explained in this book.

In Bayesian statistics, rather than considering the sample of data on its own, a "prior distribution" is set up with information that is already available. For instance, the researcher may give a numerical value and weighting to previous opinion and experience as well as previous research findings.

One consideration is that different researchers may put different weighting on the same previous findings.

The new sample data are then used to adjust this prior information to form a "posterior distribution." Thus these resulting figures have taken *both* the disparate old data *and* the new data into account.

Bayesian methodology is intuitively appealing because it reflects how we think. When we read about a new study we do not consider its results in isolation, we factor it in to our pre-existing opinions, knowledge, and experience of dealing with patients.

It is only recently that computer power has been sufficient to calculate the complex models that are needed for Bayesian analysis.

···· STATISTICS AT WORK

In this section we have given five real-life examples of how researchers use statistical techniques to describe and analyze their work.

The extracts have been taken from research papers published in the *British Medical Journal* (reproduced with permission of The BMJ Publishing Group), *The Lancet* (reproduced with permission from Elsevier), and the *New England Journal of Medicine* (reproduced with permission from Massachusetts Medical Society). If you want to see the original papers, you can download them from, respectively:

- The *BMJ* website http://www.bmj.com/

- *The Lancet* website http://www.thelancet.com/

- The *NEJM* website http://content.nejm.org/

If you wish, you can use this part to test what you have learnt:

- First, go through the abstracts and results and note down what statistical techniques have been used.

- Then try to work out why the authors have used those techniques.

- Next, try to interpret the results.

- Finally, check out your understanding by comparing it with our commentary.

The following extract is reproduced with permission from The BMJ Publishing Group.

Standard deviation, relative risk and numbers needed to treat

Alho, O.-P., Koivunen, P., Penna, T., *et al.* (2007). Tonsillectomy versus watchful waiting in recurrent streptococcal pharyngitis in adults: randomised controlled trial. *BMJ* **334**: 939. (Originally published online 8 Mar 2007; doi:10.1136/bmj.39140.632604.55.)

Abstract

Objective: To determine the short-term efficacy and safety of tonsillectomy for recurrent streptococcal pharyngitis in adults.

Design: Randomised controlled trial.

Setting: Academic referral centre in Finland.

Participants: 70 adults with documented recurrent episodes of streptococcal group A pharyngitis.

Intervention: Instant tonsillectomy (n=36) or remaining on waiting list as control (n=34).

Main outcome measures: Percentage change in the risk of an episode of streptococcal pharyngitis at 90 days. Rates of all episodes of pharyngitis and days with symptoms and adverse effects.

Results: The mean (SD) follow-up was 164 (63) days in the control group and 170 (12) days in the tonsillectomy group. At 90 days, streptococcal pharyngitis had recurred in 24% (8/34) in the control group and 3% (1/36) in the tonsillectomy group (difference 21%; 95% confidence interval 6% to 36%). The number needed to undergo tonsillectomy to prevent one recurrence was 5 (95% confidence interval 3 to 16). During the whole follow-up, the rates of other episodes of pharyngitis and days with throat pain and fever were significantly lower in the tonsillectomy group than in the control group. The most common morbidity related to tonsillectomy was postoperative throat pain (mean length 13 days, SD 4).

Conclusions: Adults with a history of documented recurrent episodes of streptococcal pharyngitis were less likely to have further streptococcal or other throat infections or days with throat pain if they had their tonsils removed.

What statistical methods were used and why?

Although tonsillectomy has been used to prevent recurrent streptococcal throat infections, a recent review showed no evidence that it was effective in adults. This randomized controlled trial on adults with recurrent episodes of streptococcal pharyngitis sought to determine the effects of tonsillectomy.

The authors assumed that the length of follow-up was *normally distributed*, so compared the two groups by giving their *mean* length of follow-up. They wanted to indicate how much the length of follow-up was spread around the mean, so gave the *standard deviation* of the number of days.

As there were different numbers of adults in each group, *percentages* were given as a scale on which to compare the number of patients with a recurrence of streptococcal pharyngitis (the *incidence* of pharyngitis).

This was a *prospective* study, following two *cohorts* of adults, and used the difference in incidences of recurrence of streptococcal pharyngitis to compare the effect of the two different methods of management.

The authors wanted to give the range that was likely to contain the true difference, so gave it with its 95% *confidence interval*.

The *null hypothesis* was that there would be no difference between the incidences of recurrence of streptococcal pharyngitis in the two groups.

What do the results mean?

The standard deviation of the mean duration of postoperative throat pain was 4 days.

In this group:

1 SD below the average is 13 − 4 = 9 days.

1 SD above the average is 13 + 4 = 17 days.

± 1 SD will include 68.2% of the subjects, so 68.2% of adults will have had postoperative throat pain for between 9 and 17 days.

95.4% had pain for between 5 and 21 days (± 2 SD).

99.7% of the patients would have had postoperative throat pain for between 1 and 25 days (± 3 SD).

8 adults out of 34 in the control group had a recurrence of streptococcal pharyngitis. As a percentage, this is:

$$\frac{8}{34} \times 100 = 24\%$$

This is the same as the risk, or probability, that a recurrence would happen in this group.

The difference in incidence between recurrences over 90 days was 21%. The confidence interval (CI) of 6% to 36% doesn't include 0% (no difference in risk), so it is statistically significant.

The risk ratio wasn't given in the abstract, but can be calculated by dividing the risk in the tonsillectomy group with that in the control group:

$$\frac{3\%}{24\%} = 0.125$$

The risk ratio of <1 shows that the rate of recurrence in the tonsillectomy group was lower than that in the control group.

From the results of the research, the clinician can calculate absolute risk reduction (ARR), number needed to treat (NNT), and relative risk reduction (RRR) from doing a tonsillectomy.

ARR = [risk in the control group] − [risk in the tonsillectomy group] = 24% − 3% = 21%

$$NNT = \frac{100}{ARR} = \frac{100}{21} = 4.8$$

So, for every 5 adults, tonsillectomy would prevent one patient from experiencing a recurrence of streptococcal pharyngitis in the first 90 days.

The risk of reactions was reduced from 24% to 3% by tonsillectomy, so the RRR is given by:

$$RRR = \frac{24\% - 3\%}{24\%} = \frac{21}{24} = 0.88 = 88\%$$

The researchers concluded that adults with recurrent episodes of streptococcal pharyngitis were less likely to have further streptococcal throat infections or days with throat pain if they had their tonsils removed.

Tonsillectomy significantly reduced rates of a recurrence of streptococcal pharyngitis in the first 90 days, with an NNT of 5.

The following extract is reproduced with permission from Elsevier.

Odds ratios and confidence intervals

Yin, P., Jiang, C.Q., Cheng, K.K., *et al.* (2007). Passive smoking exposure and risk of COPD among adults in China: the Guangzhou Biobank Cohort Study. *Lancet* **370**: 751–57.

Summary

Background: Chronic obstructive pulmonary disease (COPD) is a leading cause of mortality in China, where the population is also exposed to high levels of passive smoking, yet little information exists on the effects of such exposure on COPD. We examined the relation between passive smoking and COPD and respiratory symptoms in an adult Chinese population.

Methods: We used baseline data from the Guangzhou Biobank Cohort Study. Of 20 430 men and women over the age of 50 recruited in 2003–06, 15 379 never smokers (6497 with valid spirometry) were included in this cross-sectional analysis. We measured passive smoking exposure at home and work by two self-reported measures (density and duration of exposure). Diagnosis of COPD was based on spirometry and defined according to the GOLD guidelines.

Findings: There was an association between risk of COPD and self-reported exposure to passive smoking at home and work (adjusted odds ratio 1.48, 95% CI 1.18–1.85 for high level exposure; equivalent to 40 h a week for more than 5 years). There were significant associations between reported respiratory symptoms and increasing passive smoking exposure (1.16, 1.07–1.25 for any symptom).

What statistical methods were used and why?

The authors felt that the evidence of effects of passive smoking exposure on lung function showed mixed results.

They therefore analyzed a large *cohort* of patients to study the association between passive smoking and COPD. They studied the *odds* of COPD in passive smokers with those of patients who had not been exposed to tobacco and compared the two groups with an *odds ratio*.

The authors wanted to give the ranges that were likely to contain the true odds ratios, so gave them with their 95% *confidence intervals* (CI).

What do the results mean?

In the *Lancet* paper, the authors gave the results and odds ratios for 8 outcomes of each of the trials. We have extracted the results for COPD risk for those with the highest passive exposure to tobacco (*Table 9*).

Table 9. Relation between self-reported passive smoking exposure and COPD in never smokers: total hours of adulthood home and work exposure

	n (%) without COPD	*n* (%) with COPD	OR (95% CI)
<2 yrs of 40 h per week	2999 (94.0)	191 (6.0)	1
2–5 yrs of 40 h per week	1409 (94.5)	82 (5.5)	0.91 (0.70–1.19)
>5 yrs of 40 h per week	1660 (91.4)	156 (8.6)	1.48 (1.18–1.84)
			$P = 0.001$

Consider the risk of COPD:

Odds for COPD in patients with low passive exposure (<2 yrs) to tobacco =

$$\frac{\text{number of times the event (COPD) happens}}{\text{number of times it doesn't happen}}$$

$$= \frac{191}{2999} = 0.064$$

Odds for COPD in patients with high passive exposure (>5 yrs) to tobacco

$$= \frac{156}{1660} = 0.094$$

Odds ratio (OR) =

$$\frac{\text{Odds of COPD in patients with high tobacco exposure}}{\text{Odds of COPD in patients with low tobacco exposure}}$$

$$= \frac{0.094}{0.064} = 1.48$$

The OR of >1 indicates that the rate of COPD is increased in patients with high levels of passive smoking compared to patients with low levels.

The 95% confidence interval was calculated to be 1.18–1.85. As the CI for the odds ratio doesn't include 1 (no difference in odds), the difference between the results in this study is statistically significant.

The OR between reported respiratory symptoms and increasing passive smoking exposure was 1.16. Again, the OR of >1 indicates an increased risk with high levels of passive smoking. The fact that the CI for the OR is 1.07–1.25, and doesn't include 1, indicates that this result is also significant.

The authors concluded that exposure to passive smoking is associated with an increased prevalence of COPD and respiratory symptoms.

The following extract is reproduced with permission from The BMJ Publishing Group.

Correlation and regression

Priest, P., Yudkin, P., McNulty, C., and Mant, D. (2001). Antibacterial prescribing and antibacterial resistance in English general practice: cross sectional study. *BMJ* **323**: 1037–1041.

Abstract

Objective: To quantify the relation between community based antibacterial prescribing and antibacterial resistance in community acquired disease.

Design: Cross sectional study of antibacterial prescribing and antibacterial resistance of routine isolates within individual practices and primary care groups.

Setting: 405 general practices in south west and north west England.

Main outcome measures: Correlation between antibacterial prescribing and resistance for urinary coliforms.

Results: Antibacterial resistance in urinary coliform isolates is common but the correlation with prescribing rates was relatively low for individual practices (ampicillin and amoxicillin r_s=0.20, P=0.001). The regression coefficient was also low; a practice prescribing 20% less ampicillin and amoxicillin than average would have about 1% fewer resistant isolates.

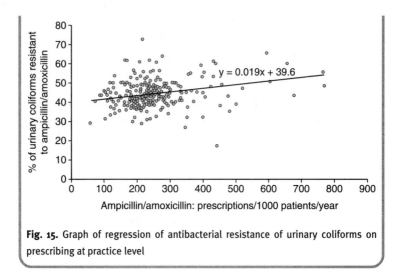

Fig. 15. Graph of regression of antibacterial resistance of urinary coliforms on prescribing at practice level

What statistical methods were used and why?

The researchers wanted to know whether there was a relationship between antibacterial prescribing and antibiotic resistance, so they needed to measure the *correlation* between the two.

As the data were *skewed*, i.e., not *normally distributed*, they needed to use the *Spearman rank correlation coefficient* as a measure of the correlation.

They wished to predict how much a 20% reduction in antibiotic prescribing would be likely to reduce antibacterial resistance. To do this they needed to calculate the *regression coefficient*.

What do the results mean?

The Spearman rank correlation coefficient for penicillin prescribing and resistance for urinary coliforms is given as $r_s = 0.20$.

The r indicates that it is the correlation coefficient, and the small s behind it shows that it is a Spearman rank correlation coefficient.

The r value of 0.20 indicates a low correlation.

$P = 0.001$ indicates that an r value of 0.20 would have happened by chance 1 in 1000 times if there were really no correlation.

Figure 15 shows the authors' *regression graph* comparing antibiotic prescribing with antibiotic resistance. Each dot represents one practice's results. The line through the dots is the *regression line*.

The authors show the *regression equation* in the graph: $y = 0.019x + 39.6$.

In this equation:

x (the horizontal axis of the graph) indicates the number of penicillin prescriptions per 1000 patients per year.

y (the vertical axis of the graph) indicates the percentage of urinary coliforms resistant to penicillin.

The *regression constant* of 39.6 is the point at which the regression line would hit the vertical axis of the graph (when number of prescriptions = 0).

The *regression coefficient* gives the slope of the line—the percentage of resistant bacteria reduces by 0.019 for every one less penicillin prescription per 1000 patients per year.

Using this value, the authors calculated that a practice prescribing 20% less penicillin than average would only have about 1% fewer resistant bacteria.

The authors therefore suggested that trying to reduce the overall level of antibiotic prescribing in UK general practice may not be the most effective strategy for reducing antibiotic resistance in the community.

The following extract is reproduced with permission from the Massachusetts Medical Society, © 2007; all rights reserved.

Survival analysis

Sjöström, L., Narbro, K., Sjöström, C.D., *et al.* (2007). Effects of bariatric surgery on mortality in Swedish obese subjects. *N Engl J Med* **357**: 741–52.

Abstract

Background: Obesity is associated with increased mortality. Weight loss improves cardiovascular risk factors, but no prospective interventional studies have reported whether weight loss decreases overall mortality. In fact, many observational studies suggest that weight reduction is associated with increased mortality.

Methods: The prospective, controlled Swedish Obese Subjects study involved 4047 obese subjects. Of these subjects, 2010 underwent bariatric surgery (surgery group) and 2037 received conventional treatment (matched control group). We report on overall mortality during an average of 10.9 years of follow-up.

Cox proportional-hazards models were used to evaluate time to death while adjusting for potentially significant risk factors.

Results: There were 129 deaths in the control group and 101 deaths in the surgery group.

The overall hazard ratio was 0.76 in the surgery group ($P = 0.04$), as compared with the control group.

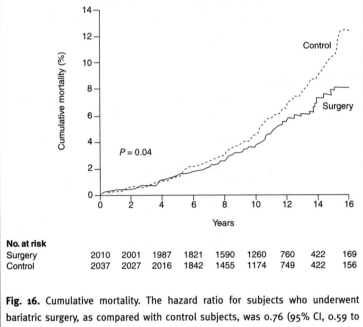

Fig. 16. Cumulative mortality. The hazard ratio for subjects who underwent bariatric surgery, as compared with control subjects, was 0.76 (95% CI, 0.59 to 0.99; *P*=0.04), with 129 deaths in the control group and 101 in the surgery group.

What statistical methods were used and why?

The authors wanted to find out whether surgical procedures to treat severe obesity (bariatric surgery) affect mortality.

The *null hypothesis* was that there was no difference between the surgery group and those receiving conventional treatment.

The *cumulative mortality plot* (*Fig. 16*) was used to give a visual representation of the mortality over time in each group. The survival between these two groups was compared with the *hazard ratio*, and the likelihood that there was no real difference between the groups was given by the *P value*.

The *Cox regression model* was used so that the effect of different variables could be studied.

What do the results mean?

The ratio of the chance (hazard) of death in the surgery group, divided by the chance of death in the conventional treatment group, was calculated to be 0.76. A hazard ratio (HR) of 1 would mean the risk is 1× that of the second group, i.e., the same. The hazard ratio of 0.76 in this study means that there was a lower risk in the surgery group.

$P = 0.04$, so the probability of the difference having happened by chance is 0.04 in 1, i.e., 1 in 25.

As $P < 0.05$, this is considered to be statistically significant.

This is stated another way by giving the 95% confidence interval, given in *Fig. 16*. The CI of 0.59 to 0.99 doesn't include 1 (no difference in risk), so again demonstrating statistical significance.

The conclusion was that bariatric surgery for severe obesity is associated with decreased overall mortality.

The following extract is reproduced with permission from The BMJ Publishing Group.

Sensitivity, specificity and predictive values

Hopper, A.D., Cross, S.S., Hurlstone, D.P., *et al.* (2007). Pre-endoscopy serological testing for coeliac disease: evaluation of a clinical decision tool. *BMJ* **334**; 729. (Originally published online 23 Mar 2007; doi:10.1136/bmj.39133.668681.BE.)

Abstract

Objective: To determine an effective diagnostic method of detecting all cases of coeliac disease in patients referred for gastroscopy without performing routine duodenal biopsy.

Design: An initial retrospective cohort of patients attending for gastroscopy was analysed to derive a clinical decision tool that could increase the detection of coeliac disease without performing routine duodenal biopsy. The tool incorporated serology and stratifying patients according to their referral symptoms ("high risk" or "low risk" of coeliac disease). The decision tool was then tested on a second cohort of patients attending for gastroscopy. In the second cohort all patients had a routine duodenal biopsy and serology performed.

Participants: 2000 consecutive adult patients referred for gastroscopy recruited prospectively.

Main outcome measure: Evaluation of a clinical decision tool using patients' referral symptoms, tissue transglutaminase antibody results, and duodenal biopsy results.

Results: No cases of coeliac disease were missed by the pre-endoscopy testing algorithm.

Evaluation of the clinical decision tool gave a sensitivity, specificity, positive predictive value, and negative predictive value of 100%, 60.8%, 9.3%, and 100%, respectively.

Table 10. Two-way table of number of patients categorised as having coeliac disease by clinical decision tool and by gold standard (duodenal biopsy): values derived from data given in the paper.

		Outcome of duodenal biopsy		Total
		Positive	Negative	
Result from clinical decision tool	Positive	77	753	830
	Negative	0	1170	1170
Total		77	1923	2000

What statistical methods were used and why?

The researchers wanted to know whether they could use their clinical decision tool to replace duodenal biopsy in diagnosing coeliac disease. They decided whether patients actually had coeliac disease by using a "gold standard" test, duodenal biopsy.

We have used a *two-way table* to show the results, shown in *Table 10*.

Sensitivity, specificity, predictive values, and *likelihood ratios* were used to give the value of their clinical decision tool.

What do the results mean?

In a perfect test, the sensitivity, specificity, and predictive values would each have a value of 1. The lower the value (the nearer to zero), the less useful the test is in that respect.

Sensitivity shows the rate of pick-up of the disease—if a patient has coeliac disease, how often the tool will be positive.

This is calculated from: $\frac{77}{77} = 1.0$, or 100%

Specificity is the rate at which the tool can exclude a coeliac disease—if the patient is in fact healthy, how often the tool will be negative.

This is given by: $\frac{1170}{1923} = 0.608$, or 60.8%

Positive predictive value is the likelihood that the patient has coeliac disease if the tool is positive.

$\frac{77}{830} = 0.093$, or 9.3%

So, in patients for whom the tool is positive, the incidence of coeliac disease is 9.3%. However, 91 in 100 patients with a positive result won't actually have coeliac disease.

Negative predictive value shows the likelihood that the patient won't have coeliac disease if the tool result is negative.

$\frac{1170}{1170} = 1.0$, or 100%

Following a negative test, no patient will turn out to have the condition.

Likelihood ratio (LR) is the likelihood that the tool result would be positive in a patient with coeliac disease, compared to the likelihood that that same result would be expected in a healthy patient.

$$LR = \frac{\text{sensitivity}}{(1 - \text{specificity})} = \frac{1}{1 - 0.608} = \frac{1}{0.392} = 2.55$$

So, if the tool is positive in a patient, that patient is 2.6 times more likely to have coeliac disease than if the tool is negative.

Pre-endoscopy serological testing in combination with biopsy of high risk cases had a 100% negative predictive value—no patients who were negative were found to have coeliac disease. The authors therefore suggested that patients with a negative result might not need a duodenal biopsy.

GLOSSARY

Cross-references to other parts of the glossary are given in *italics*.

Absolute risk reduction, ARR

The difference between the event *rate* in the intervention group and that in the control group. It is also the reciprocal of the *NNT*.

Alpha, α

The alpha value is equivalent to the *P value* and should be interpreted in the same way.

ANCOVA (ANalysis of COVAriance)

Analysis of covariance is an extension of *analysis of variance* (ANOVA) to allow for the inclusion of *continuous variables* in the model. See page 29.

ANOVA (ANalysis Of VAriance)

This is a group of statistical techniques used to compare the *means* of two of more samples to see whether they come from the same population. See page 29.

Association

A word used to describe a relationship between two *variables*.

Beta, β

The beta value is the probability of accepting a *hypothesis* that is actually false. $1 - \beta$ is known as the *power* of the study.

Bayesian statistics

An alternative way of analyzing data, it creates and combines numerical values for prior belief, existing data and new data. See page 72.

Binary variable

See *categorical variable* below.

Bimodal distribution

Where there are 2 *modes* in a set of data, it is said to be bimodal. See page 15.

Binomial distribution

When data can only take one of two values (for instance male or female), it is said to follow a binomial *distribution*.

Bonferroni

A method that allows for the problems associated with making multiple comparisons. See page 69.

Box and whisker plot

A graph showing the *median*, *range*, and *interquartile range* of a set of values. See page 13.

Case-control study

A retrospective study that investigates the relationship between a risk factor and one or more outcomes. This is done by selecting patients who already have the disease or outcome (*cases*), matching them to patients who do not (controls) and then comparing the effect of the risk factor on the two groups. Compare this with *Cohort study*. See page 40.

Cases

This usually refers to patients but could refer to hospitals, wards, counties, blood samples, etc.

Categorical variable

A *variable* whose values represent different categories of the same feature. Examples include different blood groups, different eye colors, and different ethnic groups.

When the variable has only two categories, it is termed "*binary*" (e.g., gender). Where there is some inherent ordering (e.g., mild, moderate, severe), this is called an "*ordinal*" variable.

Causation

The direct relationship of the cause to the effect that it produces, usually established in experimental studies.

Censored

A censored observation is one in which we do not have information for all of the observation period. This is usually seen in *survival analysis* in which patients are followed for some time and then move away or withdraw consent for inclusion in the study. We cannot include them in the analysis after this point as we do not know what has happened to them. See page 57.

Central tendency

The "central" scores in a set of figures. *Mean*, *median*, and *mode* are measures of central tendency.

Chi-squared test, χ^2

The chi-squared test is a test of association between two *categorical variables*. See page 34.

Cohort study

A prospective, observational study that follows a group (cohort) over a period of time and investigates the effect of a treatment or risk factor. Compare this with *case-control study*. See page 37.

Confidence interval, CI

A range of values within which we are fairly confident the true *population* value lies. For example, a 95% CI means that we can be 95% confident that the population value lies within those limits. See page 20.

Confounding

A confounding factor is the effect of a *covariate* or factor that cannot be separated out. For example, if women with a certain condition received a new treatment and men received placebo, it would not be possible to separate the treatment effect from the effect due to gender. Therefore, gender would be a confounding factor.

Continuous variable

A *variable* that can take any value within a given range, for instance, BP. Compare this with *discrete variable*.

Correlation

When there is a linear relationship between two *variables*, there is said to be a correlation between them. Examples are height and weight in children, or socioeconomic class and mortality.

Measured on a scale from −1 (perfect negative correlation), through 0 (no relationship between the variables at all), to +1 (perfect positive correlation). See page 48.

Correlation coefficient

A measure of the strength of the linear relationship between two *variables*. See page 48.

Covariate

A covariate is a *continuous variable* that is not of primary interest but is measured because it may affect the outcome and may therefore need to be included in the analysis.

Cox regression model

A method that explores the effects of different *variables* on survival. See page 60.

Database

A collection of records that is organized for ease and speed of retrieval.

Degrees of freedom, df

The number of degrees of freedom, often abbreviated to df, is the number of independent pieces of information available for the statistician to make the calculations.

Descriptive statistics

Descriptive statistics are those that describe the *data* in a *sample*. They include *means, medians, standard deviations, quartiles*, and *histograms*. They are designed to give the reader an understanding of the data. Compare this with *inferential statistics*.

Discrete variable

A *variable* in which the data can only be certain values, usually whole numbers, for example, the number of children in families. Compare this with *continuous variable*.

Distribution

A distinct pattern of data may be considered as following a distribution. Many patterns of data have been described, the most useful of which is the *normal* distribution. See page 9.

Fisher's exact test

Fisher's exact test is an accurate test for association between *categorical variables*. See page 35.

Fields

See *variables* below.

Hazard ratio, HR

The HR is the ratio of the hazard (chance of something harmful happening) of an event in one group of observations divided by the hazard of an event in a different group. An HR of 1 implies no difference in risk between the two groups, an HR of 2 implies double the risk. The HR should be stated with its *confidence intervals*. See page 61.

Histogram

A graph of *continuous* data with the data categorized into a number of classes. See example on page 15.

Hypothesis

A statement that can be tested that predicts the relationship between *variables*.

Incidence

The rate or proportion of a group developing a condition within a given period.

Inferential statistics

All statistical methods that test something are inferential. They estimate whether the results suggest that there is a real difference in the *populations*. Compare this with *descriptive statistics*.

Intention to treat

An intention to treat analysis is one in which patients are included in the analysis according to the group into which they were randomized, even if they did not actually receive the treatment.

Interaction

An interaction is when two or more *variables* are related to one another and therefore not acting independently.

Interquartile range, IQR

A measure of spread given by the difference between the first *quartile* (the value below which 25% of the cases lie) and the third quartile (the value below which 75% of the cases lie). See page 13.

Intraclass correlation coefficient

This correlation measures the *level of agreement* between two *continuous variables*. It is commonly used to look at how accurately a test can be repeated, for instance, by different people. See page 68.

Kaplan–Meier survival plot

Kaplan–Meier plots are a method of graphically displaying the survival of a sample *cohort* of which the survival estimates are recalculated whenever there is a death. See page 58.

Kappa, κ

This is a measure of the *level of agreement* between two *categorical* measures. It is often used to look at how accurately a test can be repeated, for instance, by different people. See page 67.

Kolmogorov Smirnov test

Kolmogorov Smirnov tests the hypothesis that the collected data are from a *normal distribution*. It is therefore used to assess whether *parametric* statistics can be used. See page 29.

Kruskal Wallis test

This is a *nonparametric* test which compares two or more independent groups. See page 33.

Level of agreement

A comparison of how well people or tests agree. See page 67.

Life table

A table of the proportion of patients surviving over time. It is used in survival analysis. See page 57.

Likelihood ratio, LR

This is the likelihood that a test result would be expected in patients with a condition, divided by the likelihood that that same result would be expected in patients without that condition. See page 65.

Log rank test

A *nonparametric* test used for the comparison of survival estimates with *Kaplan–Meier* or *life table* estimates. See page 59.

Logistic regression

Logistic regression is a variation of *linear regression* that is used when there are only two possible outcomes. See page 55.

Mann–Whitney U test

A *nonparametric* test to see whether there is a significant difference between two sets of data that have come from two different sets of *subjects*. See page 31.

Mantel Haenszel test

An extension of the *chi-squared* test to compare several two-way tables. This technique can be applied in *meta-analysis*. See page 36.

Mean

The sum of the observed values divided by the number of observations. Compare this with *median* and *mode*. See page 9.

Median

The middle observation when the observed values are ranked from smallest to largest. Compare this with *mean* and *mode*. See page 12.

Meta-analysis

Meta-analysis is a method of combining results from a number of independent studies to give one overall estimate of effect. See page 21 for an example.

Mode

The most commonly occurring observed value. Compare this with *mean* and *median*. See page 14.

Negative predictive value (NPV)

If a diagnostic test is negative, the NPV is the chance that a patient does not have the condition. Compare this with *positive predictive value*. See page 64.

Nominal data

Data that can be placed in named categories that have no particular order, for example, eye color.

Nonparametric test

A test which is not dependent on the *distribution* (shape) of the data. See page 31.

Normal distribution

This refers to a *distribution* of data that is symmetrical. In a graph it forms a characteristic bell shape. See page 9.

Null hypothesis

A hypothesis that there is no difference between the groups being tested. The result of the test either supports or rejects that hypothesis.

Paradoxically, the null hypothesis is usually the opposite of what we are actually interested in finding out. If we want to know whether there is a difference between two treatments, then the null hypothesis would be that there is no difference. The statistical test would be used to try to disprove this. See page 27.

Number needed to harm, NNH

NNH is the number of patients that need to be treated for one to be harmed by the treatment. See page 46.

Number needed to treat, NNT

NNT is the number of patients that need to be treated for one to get benefit. See page 43.

Odds

The ratio of the number of times an event happens to the number of time it does not happen in a group of patients. Odds and *risk* give similar values when considering rare events (e.g., winning the lottery), but may be substantially different for common events (e.g., not winning the lottery!). See page 40.

Odds ratio (OR)

The *odds* of an event happening in one group, divided by the odds of it happening in another group. See page 40.

One-tailed test

A test where the *null hypothesis* can only be rejected in one direction, for example if new treatment is worse than current treatment but not if it is better. It should only rarely be used. Compare this with a *two-tailed test*. See page 69.

Ordinal data

Data that can be allocated to categories that can be "ordered," e.g., from least to strongest. An example is the staging of malignancy.

P value

Usually used to test a *null hypothesis*, the *P* value gives the probability of any observed differences having happened by chance. See page 24.

Parametric test

Any test that has an assumption that the data needs to follow a certain distribution can be considered to be a parametric test. The most common distribution that the data need to follow is the *normal distribution*. Examples are the *t* test and *ANOVA*. See page 28.

Pearson correlation coefficient

A method of calculating a correlation coefficient if the values are sampled from a *normal* population. See page 51.

Percentage

The number of items in a category, divided by the total number in the group, then multiplied by 100. See page 7.

Poisson distribution

This *distribution* represents the number of events happening in a fixed time interval, for instance, the number of deaths in a year.

Poisson regression

A variation of *regression* calculations that allows for the frequency of rare events. See page 56.

Population

The complete set of subjects from which a sample is drawn.

Positive predictive value, PPV

If a diagnostic test is positive, the PPV is the chance that a patient has the condition. Compare this with *negative predictive value*. See page 63.

Power

The power of a study is the probability that it will detect a statistically *significant* difference. See page 71.

Prevalence

The proportion of a group with a condition at a single point in time. See page 70.

Quartiles

A *median* value may be given with its quartiles. The 1st quartile point has ¼ of the data below it, the 3rd quartile has ¾ of the data below it. See page 13.

r

Where there is a linear relationship between two variables there is said to be a *correlation* between them. The *correlation coefficient* gives the strength of that relationship. See page 48.

R^2

An estimate of the amount of the variation in the data that is being explained by a *regression* model. See page 55.

Range

The difference between the maximum and minimum score in a set of figures.

Rank

A numerical value given to an observation showing its relative order in a set of data.

Rate

The number of times that an event happens in a fixed period of time.

Regression

Regression analysis is a technique for finding the relationship between two *variables*, one of which is dependent on the other. See page 53.

Relative risk

Risk ratio is often referred to as *relative risk*. However, *odds ratios* are also a measure of relative risk.

Relative risk reduction, RRR

The proportion by which an intervention reduces the *risk* of an event. Compare this with *absolute risk reduction*. See page 43.

Risk

The probability of occurrence of an event. Calculated by dividing the number of events by the number of people at risk. See page 37.

Risk ratio, RR

The *risk* of an event happening in one group, divided by the risk of it happening in another group. See page 37.

ROC

Receiver Operator Characteristic (ROC): in a screening test, a cut-off value that gives an increase in sensitivity will give a decrease in specificity. A ROC curve is a graph showing the specificity and sensitivity for different possible values of the screening test. It helps us choose the test cut-off value that gives the best compromise between sensitivity and specificity.

Sample

A small group drawn from a larger population.

Sensitivity

This is the rate of pick-up of a condition in a test. In other words, the proportion of patients with the condition having a positive test result. See page 63. Compare this with *specificity*.

Significance

The probability of getting the results if the *null hypothesis* is true. See page 25.

Spearman rank correlation coefficient

An estimate of *correlation* used for *nonparametric variables*. See page 51.

Specificity

The rate of elimination of the possibility of disease by a test. In other words, the proportion of patients without the condition that has a negative test result. See page 63.

Skewed data

A lack of symmetry in the *distribution* of data. See page 12.

Standard deviation, SD

A measure of the spread of scores away from the *mean*. See page 16.

Standard error of the mean

A measure of how close the *sample mean* is likely to be to the *population* mean.

Stratified

A stratified *sample* is one that has been split into a number of subgroups.

Student's *t* test

See *t test.*

Subjects

The *sample* in a study.

t test (also known as Student's *t* test)

The *t* test is a *parametric* test used to compare the *means* of two groups. See page 28.

Transformation

A transformation is where a mathematical formula is used to change the data. This will often be done to try to make the data follow a *normal distribution* so that a *parametric* test can be used. See page 30.

Two-tailed test

A test where the *null hypothesis* can be rejected whether the new treatment is better or worse than the current treatment. Compare this with a *one-tailed test*. See page 69.

Type I and II errors

Any statistical test can fail in two ways. A *hypothesis* that is correct can be rejected (type I error), or a hypothesis that is incorrect can be accepted (type II error). The chance of making a type I error is the same as the *P value*.

Variable

Any characteristic that differs from subject to subject or time to time. In data analysis, variables may be called *fields* and refer to all the things recorded on the *cases*.

Variance

A measure of the spread of scores away from the mean. It is the square of the *standard deviation*.

Wilcoxon signed rank test

A *nonparametric* test for comparing the difference between paired groups, for instance before and after treatment. See page 33.

χ^2 test

The chi-squared test is a test of association between two *categorical variables*. See page 34.

Yates' continuity correction

This is an adjustment to the *chi-squared* test to improve the accuracy of the *P value*. See page 36.

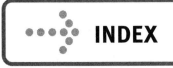

INDEX

(Page numbers in *italics* refer to the glossary)